I0106586

RING THERAPY POCKET GUIDE

For Physical, Emotional, Mental, and Spiritual

Issue - Metal Ring - Finger Placement

DR. CONSTANCE SANTEGO

MAXIMILLIAN ENTERPRISES
KELOWNA, BC

RINGS THERAPY POCKET GUIDE

Copyright © 2024 by Constance Santego.

Copy Editor & Interior Design: Constance Santego
Book Layout: ©2017 BookDesignTemplates.com
Ordering Information:
Quantity sales. Special discounts are available on quantity purchases by corporations, associations, and others. For details, contact the "Special Sales Department" at the address above.
Trade Paperback ISBN: 978-1-990062-39-1
eBook ISBN 978-1-990062-40-7
Created and published In Canada. Printed and bound in the United States of America
First Edition
Published by Maximillian Enterprises
Kelowna, BC
Canada
www.constancesantego.ca

Dedication to
My amazing teachers, friends, and clients

ALSO BY DR. CONSTANCE SANTEGO

FICTION
The Nine Spiritual Gifts Series:
Journey of a Soul – (Vol 1 Michael)
Language of a Soul – (Vol 2 Gabriel)
Prophecy of a Soul – (Vol 3 Bath Kol)
Healing of a Soul – (Vol 4 Raphael)
Miracles of a Soul – (Vol 5 Hamied)
Knowledge of a Soul – (Vol 6 Raziel)

NONFICTION
The Intuitive Life, The Gift of Prophecy, Third Edition
Fairy Tales, Dreams and Reality… Where Are You On Your
Path? Second Edition
Your Persona… The Mask You Wear
Angelic Lifestyle, A Vibrant Lifestyle
Angelic Lifestyle 42-Day Energy Cleanse
Archangel Michael's Soul Retrieval Guide
Tesla and the Future of Energy Medicine
Scaling Beyond 6 Figures: *Strategies for Health & Wellness
Professionals*
Beyond the Mind: *Harnessing the Power of Astral Projection
for Creative Awakening*
Bend, Don't Break: *Finding Your Way Back to Abundance*
Ring Therapy: *Guide to Healing and Balance*

SECRETS OF A HEALER, SERIES:
Magic Of Aromatherapy (Vol I)
Magic Of Reflexology (Vol II)
Magic Of The Gifts (Vol III)
Magic Of Muscle Testing (Vol IV)

Magic Of Iridology (Vol V)
Magic Of Massage (Vol VI)
Magic Of Hypnotherapy (Vol VII)
Magic Of Reiki (Vol VIII)
Magic Of Advanced Aromatherapy (Vol IX)
Magic Of Esthetics (Vol X)
Reiki Master's Manual (Vol XI)

ADULT COLORING JOURNALS

SERIES - ZEN COLORING:
Quantum Energy and Mindful Living Journal (Vol 1)
Reiki Energy Journal (Vol 2)
Nine Spiritual Gifts Journal (Vol 3)
I Forgive Journal (Vol 4)

SERIES – COLORING PROSPERITY:
Genie-Inspired Mandalas and Wealth Journal (Vol 1)
Entrepreneurial Mindset Reboot (Vol 2)

SERIES – HARMONIC MIND CODE:
Harmonic Mind Code Coloring Journal (Vol 1)

FOR CHILDREN
I am Big Tonight. I Don't Need the Light!

COOKBOOK
My Favorite Recipes, with a Hint of Giggle

Preface

WELCOME TO THE "RING THERAPY POCKET GUIDE," a concise and practical resource designed to help you explore the ancient wisdom of Traditional Chinese Medicine (TCM), Ayurveda, and holistic health practices. This guide focuses on the use of metal rings and finger placements to support and balance various physical, emotional, and mental conditions.

INTEGRATING TCM, AYURVEDA, AND HOLISTIC PRACTICES

- Traditional Chinese Medicine (TCM): TCM is a comprehensive medical system that has been practiced for thousands of years. It emphasizes the balance of Qi (vital energy) and the harmonious interaction of the Five Elements (Wood, Fire, Earth, Metal, and Water). This guide will delve into how TCM principles guide using metals like gold, silver, and copper to support specific organs and energy pathways.

- Ayurveda: Ayurveda, the ancient healing system from India, focuses on balancing the three doshas (Vata, Pitta, and Kapha) to achieve optimal health. This holistic approach includes diet, lifestyle, herbal remedies, and bodywork. We will explore how Ayurveda utilizes metals for their therapeutic properties and how these practices can be integrated into modern wellness routines.
- Holistic Health Practices: Holistic health practices consider the whole person— body, mind, and spirit. This guide will look at how holistic practices can be applied to using metal rings and finger placements to balance energy and support various body systems.

Purpose of This Guide

This pocket guide serves as a quick reference tool for those interested in exploring the benefits of metal therapy. By combining insights from TCM, Ayurveda, and holistic health practices, this guide provides easy access to information on how metals and their strategic placement on specific fingers can address physical, emotional, mental, and spiritual issues.

WHAT YOU WILL LEARN

- Metal Properties: Discover the unique properties and health benefits of different metals such as gold, silver, copper, titanium, and nickel.
- Finger Placement: Learn the significance of wearing metal rings on specific fingers to target various body systems and conditions.
- Quick Reference: Find fast and practical information on the appropriate metal ring and finger placement for a wide range of physical, emotional, mental, and spiritual problems.

How to Use This Guide

Each section is designed to be concise and practical, offering quick insights and actionable steps. Whether you are a holistic health practitioner or simply curious about these concepts, this guide provides valuable information that can help you enhance your well-being through the strategic use of metal rings.

Important Notice on Liability and Consulting a Doctor Disclaimer:

The information provided in this guide is intended for educational purposes only and should not be considered medical advice. The practices and suggestions described herein, including the use of metals for health purposes, are based on traditional knowledge and contemporary applications. They are not intended to diagnose, treat, cure, or prevent any disease.

> Liability: The author and publisher of this guide assume no responsibility for any adverse effects, injuries, or damages that may result from the use or misuse of the information contained herein. Readers are strongly advised to use their

own judgment and discretion when applying the practices discussed in this guide.

CONSULTING A DOCTOR: Before beginning any new health regimen, incorporating supplements, or using alternative healing practices such as those described in this guide, it is crucial to consult with a qualified healthcare provider. This is especially important for individuals with pre-existing health conditions, those who are pregnant or breastfeeding, and those currently taking medications.

SAFETY FIRST: While traditional practices offer valuable insights into health and wellness, modern medical guidance is essential to ensure your safety and well-being. Always prioritize professional medical advice and support when considering changes to your health routine.

By consulting with your healthcare provider and using this guide as a supplementary resource,

you can make informed decisions that
contribute to your overall health and well-being.

Dr. Constance Santego

Ring Therapy
Pocket Guide

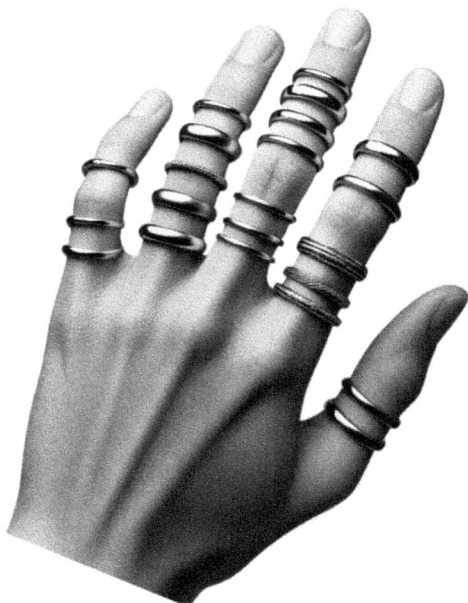

Dr. Constance Santego

Contents

Preface.. viii

Reference Chart 3

Introduction 5

    The Power of Metals and Finger
    Placement... 6

    Using This Guide..................................... 6

    Embark on Your Healing Journey........... 7

    Practical Applications: Personalized Tips
    for Muscle Testing................................. 8

    The Benefits of This Pocket Guide 8

    Why Muscle Testing Is Essential 9

    How to Perform Muscle Testing 10

Issue, Metal Ring, and Finger Placement......... 14

    Physical Issues 14

    Emotional Issues 66

    Mental Issues 70

Spiritual Issues 76

Bibliography 81

About Dr. Constance Santego 87

Reference Chart

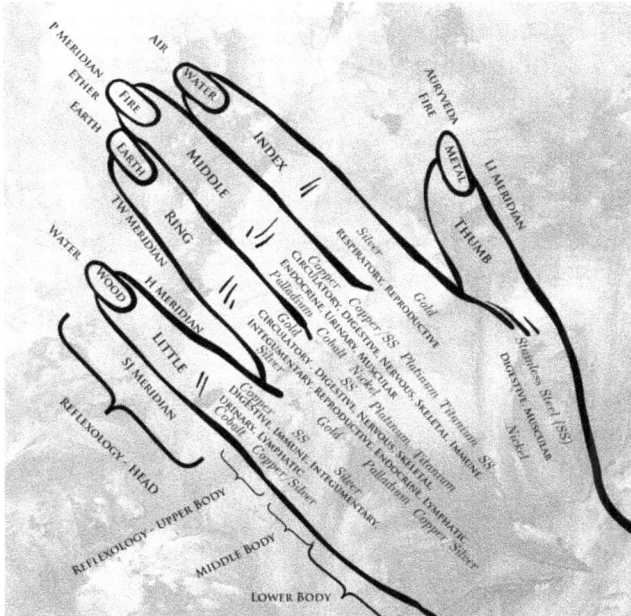

Subtle energy healing works on the principle that the body has an energy field, often referred to as the aura or biofield, which interacts with the physical, emotional, mental, and spiritual states. Practitioners believe that imbalances or blockages in this energy field can lead to illness or discomfort. Techniques such as Reiki, acupuncture, and the use of healing crystals aim to clear these blockages and restore the natural flow of energy, promoting overall well-being and facilitating the body's natural healing processes.

Ring Therapy blends the principles of subtle energy healing with the use of specific metals and strategic ring placement on fingers to influence the body's energy flow. Each metal has unique properties that can interact with the body's energy field, while the placement of rings on particular fingers corresponds to different meridians and body systems. By wearing the appropriate metal ring on the designated finger, one can help balance and direct the subtle energy, supporting physical health, emotional stability, mental clarity, and spiritual growth. This approach integrates ancient wisdom from TCM and Ayurveda, offering a holistic method to enhance well-being through the power of metals and mindful ring placement.

Introduction

In 1998, I took a class on the Five Element Theory and how to use medicinal patches to balance the body. During this class, the teacher introduced us to the fascinating practice of muscle testing metals and how they can influence our meridians. This experience sparked a profound interest in the ancient wisdom of Traditional Chinese Medicine (TCM), Ayurveda, and holistic health practices. All these years later, my journey has led me to compile this Ring Therapy Pocket Guide, a concise and practical resource for harnessing the power of metals to enhance your health and well-being.

This **Ring Therapy Pocket Guide** serves as a quick reference from the comprehensive book, **Ring Therapy: A Guide to Healing and Balance.** It distills the essential information, offering a handy guide for identifying physical, emotional, mental, and spiritual issues, along with the appropriate metal rings and finger placements. For a deeper understanding and more detailed instructions, refer to the full-length book.

The Power of Metals and Finger Placement

For centuries, various cultures have recognized the healing properties of metals and their influence on the body's energy systems. TCM and Ayurveda, in particular, have developed intricate systems that link specific metals and finger placements to different aspects of health and well-being. By understanding and applying these principles, you can harness the therapeutic benefits of metals to enhance your overall health.

Using This Guide

This pocket guide is designed to be your go-to resource for quick and practical advice. Whether you are a seasoned holistic health practitioner or new to these concepts, you will find valuable insights that can help you make informed decisions about using metal rings to support your well-being.

Embark on Your Healing Journey

Join us as we bridge the wisdom of the past with the needs of the present. Through the strategic use of metals and mindful ring placement, you can create a holistic approach to health and wellness that is both effective and empowering. Welcome to your journey of discovery and healing with the Ring Therapy Pocket Guide.

With this guide, my hope is to share the invaluable knowledge I have gained over the years, allowing you to explore and benefit from the therapeutic potential of metals. Together, let's embark on a journey towards balanced health and harmony.

Practical Applications: Personalized Tips for Muscle Testing

One of the most powerful aspects of this Ring Therapy Pocket Guide is its ability to provide practical, actionable steps for enhancing your health through the use of metal rings. This guide offers a wealth of information on the general properties of different metals and their associated finger placements for addressing various physical, emotional, mental, and spiritual conditions. However, to achieve the most precise and effective results, personalized muscle testing is recommended.

The Benefits of This Pocket Guide

This pocket guide serves as a quick reference tool, offering:

- Immediate Guidance: Find fast and accurate information about which metals and finger placements are generally beneficial for specific conditions.

- Broad Applicability: Covers a wide range of common issues, providing a solid starting point for exploring the benefits of metal therapy.
- Holistic Insights: Combines principles from TCM, Ayurveda, and holistic health practices, giving you a well-rounded understanding of how metals can influence your well-being.

Why Muscle Testing Is Essential

While the recommendations in this guide are based on traditional knowledge and modern holistic practices, every individual's body and energy system are unique. Muscle testing, also known as applied kinesiology, is a technique that can help you identify the specific metal and finger placement that will be most effective for your individual situation. Here's why muscle testing is beneficial:

- Personalized Results: Muscle testing tailors the recommendations to your unique energy and health needs, ensuring that you get the most accurate and beneficial results.
- Dynamic Adjustments: As your health and energy levels change over time, muscle testing allows you to adjust the metals and placements accordingly, maintaining optimal balance and effectiveness.
- Enhanced Precision: By pinpointing the exact metal and finger placement for your current condition, muscle testing maximizes the therapeutic benefits and minimizes any potential mismatches or ineffectiveness.

How to Perform Muscle Testing

To conduct muscle testing and determine the most effective metal and finger placement for your needs, follow these steps:

1. Preparation:
   - Find a quiet, comfortable space free from distractions.
   - Hydrate well and ensure you are in a calm, relaxed state.
2. Establishing a Baseline:
   - A simple statement, such as "My name is [Your Name]," establishes a baseline response. This will help you understand your body's natural resistance and strength.
3. Testing Metals:
   - Hold a piece of the metal you wish to test in your hand.
   - Make a clear, direct statement such as "Gold is beneficial for my [specific condition]."
   - Observe the muscle response—if the muscle remains strong, the metal is likely beneficial; if it weakens, it may not be suitable.
4. Testing Finger Placements:
   - Place the chosen metal ring on different fingers and repeat the

muscle testing process for each finger placement.
- o Determine which finger placement yields the strongest and most positive muscle response.

By using this pocket guide in conjunction with muscle testing, you can create a highly personalized and effective approach to metal therapy. This combination allows you to tap into the ancient wisdom of TCM, Ayurveda, and holistic health practices while tailoring the application to your unique needs, ensuring the best possible outcomes for your health and well-being.

For more comprehensive information and an in-depth exploration of metal therapy, including detailed explanations of TCM, Ayurveda, and holistic health practices, be sure to read the first book in this series, *"Ring Therapy: A Guide to Healing and Balance."* This foundational text provides a deeper understanding of the principles and techniques that underpin this pocket guide, offering a complete framework for achieving optimal health and balance through the strategic use of metal rings.

Issue, Metal Ring, and Finger Placement

Physical Issues

PHYSICAL ISSUE	METAL RING	FINGER PLACEMENT
Abdominal Cramps	Copper Stainless Steel	*Middle or Little *Thumb or Ring or Middle
Abscess	Stainless Steel	Little or Middle

"Muscle Testing will determine the precise metal ring and finger placement tailored to your body."

Aches	Platinum	Ring or Middle
Achilles Tendon Rupture	Nickel	Thumb
Acne	Silver	Ring
Addictions	Platinum	Ring or Middle
Addison's Disease	Palladium	Ring
Adenoids	Silver	Index
Adrenal Problems	Palladium	Middle
Aging Problem	Silver	Ring or Little
AIDS	Stainless Steel	Little or Middle
Alcoholism	Platinum	Ring or Middle

Allergies	Stainless Steel	Index
Alzheimer's	Platinum	Thumb
Amenorrhea	Gold	Ring or Index
Andropause (Male Menopause)	Palladium	Ring
Anemia	Copper	Middle
Ankylosing Spondylitis	Titanium	Index
Anorectal Bleeding	Copper Stainless Steel	*Middle or Little *Thumb or Ring or Middle
Anorexia Nervosa	Copper	Middle

"Muscle Testing will determine the precise metal ring and finger placement tailored to your body."

Appendicitis	Copper Stainless Steel	*Middle or Little *Thumb or Ring or Middle
Appetite	Copper Stainless Steel	*Middle or Little *Thumb or Ring or Middle
Arrhythmia	Gold	Ring
Arteries	Gold Copper	Ring Middle
Arthritis	Copper	Index
Asphyxiating Attack	Silver	Index

Asthma	Silver	Little
Athlete's Foot	Silver	Ring or Little
Backache	Copper or Nickel	Middle
Bacterial Infections	Silver	Index
Bad Breath	Copper Stainless Steel	*Middle or Little *Thumb or Ring or Middle
Balance *(loss of)*	Platinum	Ring or Middle
Baldness	Silver	Ring or Little
Bed Sores	Silver	Ring
Bed-wetting	Gold	Ring or Index

"Muscle Testing will determine the precise metal ring and finger placement tailored to your body."

Bee Sting	Silver	Ring
Belching	Copper Stainless Steel	*Middle or Little *Thumb or Ring or Middle
Bell's Palsy	Platinum	Ring or Middle
Bladder Infections	Cobalt	Index
Bleeding Gums	Copper Stainless Steel	*Middle or Little *Thumb or Ring or Middle
Blisters	Silver	Ring or Little
Blood	Gold Copper	Ring Middle

Blood Pressure	Silver	Index
Body Odor	Silver	Ring or Little
Boils	Silver	Ring or Little
Bones	Titanium	Middle or Ring
Bone Fractures	Titanium	Middle
Bowels	Copper Stainless Steel	*Middle or Little *Thumb or Ring or Middle
Brain	Platinum	Ring or Middle
Breast Cancer	Gold	Thumb
Breathing Problems	Silver	Index

"Muscle Testing will determine the precise metal ring and finger placement tailored to your body."

Bright's Disease	Gold	Ring
	Copper	Middle
Bronchitis	Silver	Little
Bruises	Gold	Ring
	Copper	Middle
Bulimia	Copper	*Middle or Little
	Stainless Steel	*Thumb or Ring or Middle
Bunions	Titanium	Middle or Ring
Burns	Silver	Ring or Little
Bursitis	Copper	Index
	Nickel	Thumb
Buttocks	Nickel	Thumb or Middle

Cancer	Platinum	Thumb
Candida	Silver	Index
Canker Sore	Silver	Index
Car Sickness	Copper	Middle
Carbuncle	Silver	Ring
Cardiomyopathy	Gold	Ring
Carpal-Tunnel	Copper Nickel	Index Middle
Cataracts	Silver	Index
Celiac	Copper	Middle
Cellulite	Copper	Ring

"Muscle Testing will determine the precise metal ring and finger placement tailored to your body."

Cerebral Palsy	Platinum	Thumb
Chickenpox	Silver	Ring
Chills	Gold	Ring
Chronic Fatigue (CFS)	Gold	Ring
Cholesterol	Gold	Ring
Circulatory Problems	Copper	Middle
Cirrhosis	Copper	Middle
Cold Sores	Silver	Index
Colic	Copper	Middle
Colitis	Copper	Middle

Colon	Copper	Middle
Coma	Platinum	Thumb
Common Cold	Silver	Index
Compartment Syndrome	Nickel	Thumb
Congenital Adrenal Hyperplasia	Palladium	Middle
Congestion	Silver	Little
Congestive Heart Failure (CHF)	Gold	Ring
Conjunctivitis	Silver	Index
Constipation	Copper	Middle
Corns & Calluses	Copper	Ring

"Muscle Testing will determine the precise metal ring and finger placement tailored to your body."

Cortisol Imbalance	Palladium	Ring
Coughs	Silver	Little
Cramps	Copper	Middle
Crohn's Disease	Copper	Index
Croup	Silver	Little
Cushing's Disease	Palladium	Ring
Cuts	Silver	Ring
Cyst(s)	Gold	Ring
Cystic Fibrosis	Silver	Little
Cystitis	Cobalt	Index

Dandruff	Silver	Ring
Deafness	Silver	Index
Dementia	Platinum	Thumb
Dermatitis	Silver	Ring
Dermatomyositis	Nickel	Thumb
Diabetes	Palladium	Middle
Diarrhea	Copper	Middle
Diverticulitis	Copper	Index
Dizziness	Platinum	Thumb
Dry Eye	Silver	Index

"Muscle Testing will determine the precise metal ring and finger placement tailored to your body."

Dupuytren's Contracture	Nickel	Finger that is affected
Dysentery	Copper	Middle
Dysmenorrhea	Gold	Ring
Dysphagia *(Difficulty Swallowing)*	Copper	Index
Dyspnea (Shortness of Breath)	Silver	Little
Dystonia	Platinum	Thumb
Ear Problems	Silver	Index
Earache	Silver	Index
Ecchymoses	Copper	Middle
Edema	Copper	Little

Emphysema	Silver	Little
Endocarditis	Silver	Middle
Endometriosis	Gold	Ring
Epilepsy	Platinum	Thumb
Epstein-Barr Virus	Silver	Index
Erectile Dysfunction	Gold	Ring
Esophagitis	Copper	Index
Essential Tremor	Platinum	Thumb
Exzema	Silver	Ring
Eye Problems	Silver	Index

"Muscle Testing will determine the precise metal ring and finger placement tailored to your body."

Eye Strain	Silver	Index
Fainting	Platinum	Thumb
Fat	Copper	Middle
Fatigue	Gold	Ring
Fever	Silver	Index
Fibroids	Gold	Ring
Fibromyalgia	Copper or Palladium	Middle
Fistula	Copper	Middle
Flatulence	Copper	Middle
Flu (Influenza)	Silver	Index

Folliculitis	Silver	Ring
Food Poisoning	Copper	Middle
Fractures	Titanium	Middle
Frozen Shoulder	Copper	Index
Furuncle	Silver	Ring
Fungal Infections	Silver	Ring
Gallbladder Problems	Copper	Middle
Gallstones	Copper	Middle
Gangrene	Copper	Little
Gas	Copper	Middle

"Muscle Testing will determine the precise metal ring and finger placement tailored to your body."

Gastritis	Copper	Middle
Gastroenteritis	Copper	Index
Gastroesophageal Reflux Disease (GERD)	Copper	Index
Genitals	Gold	Ring
Glands	Copper	Middle
Glandular Fever	Silver	Index
Glandular Problems	Copper	Middle
Glaucoma	Silver	Index
Globus Hystericus	Platinum	Thumb
Goiter	Copper or Palladium	Middle

Gonorrhea	Gold	Ring
Gout	Copper	Index
Graves' Disease	Palladium	Ring
Grey Hair	Copper	Ring
Growths	Copper	Ring
Growth Hormone Deficiency	Palladium	Middle
Guillain-Barré	Platinum	Thumb
Gum Disease (Periodontitis)	Silver	Index
Gynecomastia	Gold	Ring
Hair Loss (Alopecia)	Copper	Ring

"Muscle Testing will determine the precise metal ring and finger placement tailored to your body."

Halitosis *(Bad Breath)*	Silver	Index
Hashimoto's Thyroiditis	Palladium	Middle
Hay Fever *(Allergic Rhinitis)*	Stainless Steel	Index
Headache	Platinum	Thumb
Hearing Loss	Silver	Index
Heart Disease	Gold	Ring
Heartburn	Copper	Middle
Hemorrhoids	Copper	Middle
Hepatitis	Copper	Middle
Herpes	Silver	Index
Hip Problems	Copper	Index

Hirsutism	Gold	Ring
Hives	Silver	Ring
Hodgkin's Disease	Silver	Index
Holding Fluids	Copper	Little
Huntington's Disease	Platinum	Thumb
Hyperactivity	Silver	Middle
Hyperglycemia	Palladium	Ring
Hyperpituitarism	Palladium	Ring

"Muscle Testing will determine the precise metal ring and finger placement tailored to your body."

Hypertension *(High Blood Pressure)*	Silver	Index
Hyperthyroidism	Palladium	Ring
Hyperventilation	Silver	Little
Hypoglycemia	Palladium	Middle
Hypopituitarism	Palladium	Middle
Hypothyroidism	Palladium	Middle
Hysterectomy	Gold	Ring
Impetigo	Silver	Ring
Impotence	Gold	Ring
Incontinence	Cobalt	Index

Indigestion	Copper	Middle
Infection	Silver	Index
Infertility	Gold	Ring
Inflammation	Copper	Index
Influenza	Silver	Index
Ingrown Toenail	Silver	Ring
Injury	Copper	Index
Insect Bite	Silver	Ring
Insomnia	Platinum	Thumb
Intestine Problems	Copper	Middle
Irritable Bowel (IBS)	Copper	Middle

"Muscle Testing will determine the precise metal ring and finger placement tailored to your body."

Iron Deficiency Anemia	Copper	Middle
Ischemia	Gold	Ring
Itchy	Silver	Ring
Jaundice	Copper	Middle
Jaw Fracture	Titanium	Middle
Jaw Pain (TMJ Disorder)	Copper	Index
Jejunitis	Copper	Middle
Jet Lag	Platinum	Thumb
Jock Itch (Tinea Cruris)	Silver	Ring
Joint Effusion (Fluid in the Joint)	Copper	Index

Joint Pain (Arthralgia)	Copper	Index
Juvenile Diabetes (Type 1 Diabetes)	Copper	Middle
Juvenile Rheumatoid Arthritis (JRA)	Copper	Index
Kawasaki Disease	Gold	Ring
Kidney Problems	Cobalt	Index
Kidney Stones	Cobalt	Index
Keratitis	Silver	Index
Keratoconus	Silver	Index
Keratoderma (Palmoplantar Keratoderma)	Silver	Ring
Keratosis Pilaris	Silver	Ring

"Muscle Testing will determine the precise metal ring and finger placement tailored to your body."

Kidney Infection *(Pyelonephritis)*	Cobalt	Index
Kidney Stones	Cobalt	Index
Klinefelter Syndrome	Gold or Palladium	Ring
Knee Pain	Copper	Index
Kyphosis	Titanium	Middle
Lactose Intolerance	Copper	Middle
Laryngitis	Silver	Little
Leprosy	Silver	Ring
Leukemia	Silver	Thumb
Leukorrhea	Gold	Ring

Lichen Planus	Silver	Ring
Liver Problems	Copper	Middle
Lockjaw	Copper	Index
Lou Gehrig's Disease	Platinum	Thumb
Low Blood Pressure (*Hypotension*)	Gold	Ring
Lungs	Silver	Little
Lupus	Silver	Index
Lyme Disease	Silver	Index
Lymphedema	Copper	Little
Lymphoma	Silver	Index

"Muscle Testing will determine the precise metal ring and finger placement tailored to your body."

Malaria	Silver	Index
Mastitis	Copper	Middle
Mastoiditis	Silver	Index
Measles	Silver	Index
Mellitus	Copper	Middle
Meniere's Disease	Silver	Index
Meningitis	Platinum	Thumb
Menopause & Perimenopausal Problems	Gold or Palladium	Ring
Menstrual Problems	Gold or Palladium	Ring
Migraine	Platinum	Thumb

Miscarriage	Gold	Ring
Mitral Valve Prolapse	Gold	Ring
Mononucleosis	Silver	Index
Motion Sickness	Platinum	Thumb
Mouth Problems	Silver	Index
Mucus Colon	Copper	Middle
Multiple Sclerosis (MS)	Platinum	Thumb
Mumps	Palladium	Ring
Muscle Problems	Nickel	Index or Thumb
Muscle Atrophy	Nickel	Thumb

"Muscle Testing will determine the precise metal ring and finger placement tailored to your body."

Muscle Cramps	Copper	Index
Muscle Strain	Nickel	Middle
Muscular Dystrophy	Nickel	Index
Myalgic Encephalomyelitis (Chronic Fatigue)	Gold	Ring
Myasthenia Gravis	Platinum	Thumb
Myocardial Infarction (Heart Attack)	Gold	Ring
Myofascial Pain Syndrome	Nickel	Middle
Myopia (Nearsightedness)	Silver	Middle
Nail Problems	Silver	Ring

Narcolepsy	Platinum	Thumb
Nasal Polyps	Silver	Little
Nausea	Copper	Middle
Neck Problems	Copper	Index
Nephritis	Cobalt	Index
Nerves	Platinum	Thumb
Neuralgia	Platinum	Thumb
Neuritis	Platinum	Thumb
Neuropathy	Platinum	Thumb
Night Blindness	Silver	Index

"Muscle Testing will determine the precise metal ring and finger placement tailored to your body."

Nodule *(Thyroid)*	Copper	Middle
Nose Problems	Silver	Little
Nosebleeds *(Epistaxis)*	Silver	Little
Numbness	Platinum	Thumb
Obesity	Copper	Middle
Oily Skin	Silver	Ring
Oral Thrush	Silver	Index
Osteoarthritis	Copper	Index
Osteomalacia	Titanium	Middle
Osteomyelitis	Titanium	Middle

Osteoporosis	Titanium	Middle
	Palladium	Middle
Otitis Externa *(Swimmer's Ear)*	Silver	Index
Otitis Media *(Middle Ear Infection)*	Silver	Index
Ovarian Cysts	Gold	Ring
Paget's Disease	Titanium	Middle
Pain	Platinum	Thumb
Palsy	Platinum	Thumb
Pancreas Problems	Copper	Middle
Pancreatitis	Copper	Middle
Paralysis	Platinum	Thumb

"Muscle Testing will determine the precise metal ring and finger placement tailored to your body."

Parasites	Copper	Middle
Parathyroid Problems	Palladium	Ring
Paresthesia	Platinum	Thumb
Parkinson's Disease	Platinum	Thumb
Peptic Ulcer	Copper	Middle
Periodontitis	Silver	Index
Peripheral Neuropathy	Platinum	Thumb
Petit Mal	Platinum	Thumb
Pfeiffer's Disease	Silver	Index
Phlebitis	Copper	Little

Piles	Copper	Middle
Pimples	Silver	Ring
Pink Eye	Silver	Index
Pituitary Gland	Gold or Palladium	Ring
Plantar Fasciitis	Nickel	Middle
Plantar Wart	Silver	Ring
Pneumonia	Silver	Little
Prolactinoma	Palladium	Ring
Polymyositis	Nickel	Middle
Poison Ivy	Silver	Ring

"Muscle Testing will determine the precise metal ring and finger placement tailored to your body."

Poison Oak	Silver	Ring
Polio	Platinum	Thumb
Polycystic Ovary Syndrome *(PCOS)*	Palladium	Ring
Polyps	Copper	Middle
Postnasal Drip	Silver	Little
Premenstrual Problems	Gold	Ring
Prostate	Gold	Ring
Prostatitis	Gold	Ring
Pruritis	Silver	Ring
Psoriasis	Silver	Ring

Psoriatic Arthritis	Copper	Index
Pyelonephritis	Cobalt	Index
Pyorrhea	Silver	Index
Q Fever	Silver	Index
Quadriceps Strain	Copper	Index
Quadriplegia	Platinum	Thumb
Quick Pulse *(Tachycardia)*	Silver	Middle
Quinsy *(Peritonsillar Abscess)*	Silver	Little
Quivering *(Tremors)*	Platinum	Thumb

"Muscle Testing will determine the precise metal ring and finger placement tailored to your body."

Rabies	Platinum	Thumb
Rash	Silver	Ring
Raynaud's	Gold	Ring
Rectum Problems	Copper	Middle
Respiratory Problems	Silver	Little
Restless Leg Syndrome	Platinum	Thumb
Retinal Detachment	Silver	Index
Rhabdomyolysis	Nickel	Middle
Rheumatic Fever	Gold	Ring
Rheumatoid Arthritis	Copper	Index

Rhinitis *(Hay Fever)*	Stainless Steel	Index
Rickets/Osteomalacia	Titanium	Middle
Ringworm *(Tinea)*	Silver	Ring
Root Canal	Silver	Index
Rosacea	Silver	Ring
Rotator Cuff Injury	Copper / Nickel	Index / Thumb
Sagging Lines	Silver	Ring
Scabies	Silver	Ring
Sciatica	Platinum	Thumb
Scleroderma	Silver	Ring

"Muscle Testing will determine the precise metal ring and finger placement tailored to your body."

Scoliosis	Titanium	Middle
Scratches	Silver	Ring
Seasickness	Platinum	Thumb
Sebaceous Cysts	Silver	Ring
Seborrhea	Silver	Ring
Senility	Platinum	Thumb
Shin Splints	Nickel	Middle
Shingles	Silver	Index
Sickle Cell Anemia	Copper	Middle
Sinus Problems	Silver	Little

Sinusitis	Silver	Little
Skeletal Problems	Titanium	Middle
Skin Cancer	Silver	Ring
Skin Problems	Silver	Ring
Skin Rash	Silver	Ring
Sleep Apnea	Silver	Little
Slipped Disc	Titanium	Middle
Smoking	Silver	Little
Snoring	Silver	Little
Solar Plexus	Copper	Middle

"Muscle Testing will determine the precise metal ring and finger placement tailored to your body."

Sores	Silver	Ring
Sore Throat (Pharyngitis)	Silver	Little
Spasms	Copper	Index
Spastic Colitis	Copper	Middle
Spider Bites	Silver	Ring
Spinal Problems	Titanium	Middle
Spleen Problems	Copper	Middle
Sprains and Strains	Copper or Nickel	Index
Sterility	Gold	Ring
Stiff Neck	Copper	Index

Stiffness	Copper	Index
Stomach Problems	Copper	Middle
Stomach Ulcers	Copper	Middle
Stroke	Platinum	Thumb
Stuttering	Platinum	Thumb
Sty	Silver	Index
Sunburn	Silver	Ring
Swelling	Copper	Little
Syphilis	Silver	Index

"Muscle Testing will determine the precise metal ring and finger placement tailored to your body."

Systemic Lupus Erythematosus *(SLE)*	Silver	Index
Tachycardia	Gold	Ring
Tapeworm	Copper	Middle
Teeth Problems	Silver	Index
Temporomandibular Joint Disorder *(TMJ)*	Copper Nickel	Index Middle
Tendonitis	Copper Nickel	Index Thumb
Testicle Problems	Gold	Ring
Tetanus	Platinum	Thumb
Throat Problems	Silver	Little

Thrombophlebitis	Copper	Little
Thrush	Silver	Index
Thymus Problems	Silver	Index
Thyroid Problems	Copper	Middle
	Palladium	Middle
Tics/Twitches	Platinum	Thumb
Tinnitus	Silver	Index
Tongue Problems	Silver	Index
Tonsillitis	Silver	Little
Tooth Decay	Silver	Index
Toxoplasmosis	Silver	Index

"Muscle Testing will determine the precise metal ring and finger placement tailored to your body."

Trichomoniasis	Gold	Ring
Trigger Finger	Nickel	Thumb
Tuberculosis *(TB)*	Silver	Little
Tumors	Gold	Ring
Turner Syndrome	Palladium	Middle
Ulcer *(Peptic)*	Copper	Middle
Ulcerative Colitis	Copper	Middle
Umbilical Hernia	Titanium	Middle
Under Weight *(Weight Loss)*	Gold	Ring
Upper Respiratory Tract Infection	Silver	Little

Urethritis	Cobalt	Index
Urinary Tract Infection (UTI)	Cobalt	Index
Urolithiasis (Kidney Stones)	Cobalt	Index
Urticaria (Hives)	Silver	Ring
Uterine Fibroids	Gold	Ring
Uterus Problems	Gold	Ring
Uveitis	Silver	Index
Vaginitis	Gold	Ring
Varicella	Silver	Index
Varicocele	Gold	Ring

"Muscle Testing will determine the precise metal ring and finger placement tailored to your body."

Varicose Veins	Copper	Little
Vasculitis	Copper	Little
Vasovagal Attack	Platinum	Thumb
Venous Thromboembolism (VTE)	Copper	Little
Vertigo	Platinum	Thumb
Viral Infections	Silver	Index
Vitiligo	Silver	Ring
Vomiting	Copper	Middle
Vulvodynia	Gold	Ring
Vulvovaginal Candidiasis	Gold	Ring

Warts	Silver	Ring
Weakness	Platinum	Thumb
Wegener's Granulomatosis	Silver	Index
Wheezing	Silver	Little
Whiplash	Copper	Index
Whooping Cough (Pertussis)	Silver	Little
Wilson's Disease	Copper	Middle
Wolff-Parkinson-White Syndrome	Gold	Ring
Worms	Copper	Middle
Wound Healing	Silver	Ring

"Muscle Testing will determine the precise metal ring and finger placement tailored to your body."

Wrinkles	Silver	Ring
Wrist Pain	Copper	Index
Xanthelasma	Silver	Ring
Xanthinuria	Copper	Index
Xanthoma	Silver	Ring
Xeroderma	Silver	Ring
Xerophthalmia	Silver	Index
Xerosis	Silver	Ring
Xerostomia *(Dry Mouth)*	Silver	Index
Yamaguchi Syndrome	Gold	Ring

Yeast Infection	Gold	Ring
Yellow Fever	Silver	Index
Yellow Nail Syndrome	Silver	Ring
Yersinia Enterocolitica Infection	Silver	Middle
Yersiniosis	Silver	Middle
Yolk Sac Tumor	Gold	Ring
Yttrium Exposure *(Toxicity)*	Copper	Middle
Yusho Disease	Copper	Middle
Zenker's Diverticulum	Copper	Middle

"Muscle Testing will determine the precise metal ring and finger placement tailored to your body."

Zika Virus	Silver	Index
Zollinger–Ellison Syndrome	Copper	Middle
Zoonotic Diseases	Silver	Index
Zoster *(Shingles)*	Silver	Index
Zygomycosis	Silver	Index

Emotional Issues

EMOTIONAL ISSUE	METAL RING	FINGER PLACEMENT
Anger	Copper	Index
Anxiety	Silver	Middle
Apathy	Platinum	Ring or Middle
Bitterness	Copper	Index
Boredom	Gold	Ring
Confusion	Platinum	Thumb
Crying	Silver	Little
Depression	Platinum	Thumb
Despair	Silver	Little
Disappointment	Platinum	Thumb

"Muscle Testing will determine the precise metal ring and finger placement tailored to your body."

Discouragement	Platinum	Thumb
Doubt	Gold	Ring
Embarrassment	Silver	Middle
Envy	Copper	Index
Exhaustion	Platinum	Thumb
Fear	Gold	Ring
Fretfulness	Silver	Middle
Frigidity	Gold	Ring
Frustration	Silver	Middle
Grief	Silver	Little
Guilt	Gold	Ring
Helplessness	Platinum	Thumb
Hopelessness	Platinum	Thumb
Hyperactivity	Silver	Little
Hysteria	Silver	Little
Impatience	Copper	Index

Inadequacy	Silver	Middle
Insecurity	Silver	Middle
Irrationality	Platinum	Thumb
Irritability	Copper	Index
Isolation	Gold	Ring
Jealousy	Copper	Index
Loneliness	Gold	Ring
Melancholy	Silver	Little
Mood Swings	Platinum	Ring or Middle
Nail Biting	Platinum	Thumb
Nervousness	Silver	Middle
Numbness	Platinum	Ring or Middle
Overthinking	Gold	Ring
Overwhelm	Platinum	Thumb
Pain	Copper	Index
Panic	Silver	Little

"Muscle Testing will determine the precise metal ring and finger placement tailored to your body."

Pessimism	Silver	Little
Procrastination	Copper	Index
Regret	Copper	Index
Remorse	Gold	Ring
Resentment	Copper	Index
Restlessness	Silver	Middle
Sadness	Silver	Little
Self-doubt	Gold	Ring
Shame	Silver	Middle
Stress	Silver	Middle
Worry	Silver	Middle

Mental Issues

MENTAL ISSUE	METAL RING	FINGER PLACEMENT
Addiction	Platinum	Thumb
Agitation	Silver	Middle
Alzheimer's	Platinum	Thumb
Attention Deficit Hyperactivity Disorder (ADHD)	Platinum	Thumb
Autism Spectrum Disorder (ASD)	Silver	Little

"Muscle Testing will determine the precise metal ring and finger placement tailored to your body."

Bipolar Disorder	Platinum	Thumb
Body Dysmorphic Disorder	Silver	Middle
Brain Fog	Platinum	Thumb
Burnout	Platinum	Thumb
Confusion	Platinum	Thumb
Delirium	Platinum	Thumb
Delusional Disorder	Platinum	Thumb
Dementia	Platinum	Thumb

Difficulty Concentrating	Platinum	Thumb
Disorientation	Platinum	Thumb
Dissociative Identity Disorder (DID)	Platinum	Thumb
Eating Disorders (Anorexia, Bulimia)	Copper	Middle
Hallucinations	Platinum	Thumb
Hoarding Disorder	Platinum	Thumb
Hysteria	Silver	Middle

"Muscle Testing will determine the precise metal ring and finger placement tailored to your body."

Insanity	Platinum	Thumb
Irritability	Silver	Middle
Lack of Focus	Platinum	Thumb
Memory Loss	Platinum	Thumb
Mental Fatigue	Platinum	Thumb
Mental Paralysis	Platinum	Thumb
Mood Swings	Platinum	Thumb
Nervous Breakdown	Platinum	Thumb
Obsessive-Compulsive Disorder (OCD)	Platinum	Thumb

Panic Disorder	Silver	Little
Paranoia	Platinum	Thumb
Phobias	Silver	Little
Psychosis	Platinum	Thumb
Post-Traumatic Stress Disorder *(PTSD)*	Silver	Middle
Psychiatric Illness	Platinum	Thumb
Psychosis	Platinum	Thumb
Racing Thoughts	Platinum	Thumb

"Muscle Testing will determine the precise metal ring and finger placement tailored to your body."

Restlessness	Platinum	Thumb
Schizophrenia	Platinum	Thumb
Sleep Disorders (Insomnia, Sleep Apnea)	Platinum	Thumb
Social Anxiety Disorder	Silver	Middle
Stress-Induced Mental Fatigue	Silver	Middle
Suicidal Thoughts	Platinum	Thumb

Spiritual Issues

SPIRITUAL ISSUE	METAL RING	FINGER PLACEMENT
Detachment from Spiritual Community	Copper	Index
Disbelief in Higher Power	Silver	Little
Disconnection from Intuition	Silver	Little
Disconnection from Source	Platinum	Thumb
Fear of Death	Gold	Ring
Fear of Spiritual Judgment	Gold	Ring

"Muscle Testing will determine the precise metal ring and finger placement tailored to your body."

Fear of the Unknown	Gold	Ring
Feeling Disconnected from Nature	Silver	Middle
Feeling Spiritually Blocked	Copper	Index
Feeling Spiritually Lost	Platinum	Middle
Feeling Spiritually Stagnant	Platinum	Thumb
Feeling Unloved by the Divine	Silver	Little
Feeling Unworthy	Gold	Ring
Inner Conflict	Silver	Middle

Inner Turmoil	Silver	Middle
Lack of Faith	Silver	Little
Lack of Gratitude	Gold	Middle
Lack of Inner Peace	Silver	Middle
Lack of Purpose	Gold	Ring
Lack of Self-Compassion	Gold	Ring
Lack of Spiritual Awareness	Platinum	Thumb
Lack of Spiritual Growth	Copper	Index
Lack of Trust in the Universe	Silver	Little

"Muscle Testing will determine the precise metal ring and finger placement tailored to your body."

Loss of Spiritual Path	Gold	Ring
Resentment toward Higher Power	Copper	Index
Spiritual Anguish	Platinum	Thumb
Spiritual Apathy	Platinum	Middle
Spiritual Confusion	Platinum	Thumb
Spiritual Despair	Platinum	Thumb
Spiritual Isolation	Copper	Index

"

Bibliography

BOOKS
Ayurveda and Metals:

- Lad, Vasant. The Complete Book of Ayurvedic Home Remedies. Harmony Books, 1999.
- Dash, Bhagwan, and Lalitesh Kashyap. Materia Medica of Ayurveda. B. Jain Publishers, 1980.

Traditional Chinese Medicine (TCM):

- Kaptchuk, Ted J. The Web That Has No Weaver: Understanding Chinese Medicine. McGraw-Hill, 2000.
- Maciocia, Giovanni. The Foundations of Chinese Medicine: A Comprehensive Text for Acupuncturists and Herbalists. Elsevier Health Sciences, 2005.

"

Holistic Health and Metal Therapy:

- Weil, Andrew. Spontaneous Healing: How to Discover and Enhance Your Body's Natural Ability to Maintain and Heal Itself. Knopf, 1995.
- Gerber, Richard. Vibrational Medicine: The #1 Handbook of Subtle-Energy Therapies. Bear & Company, 2001.

Metals in Modern Medicine:

- Andrews, P. C. Medicinal Inorganic Chemistry. Royal Society of Chemistry, 2010.
- Sigel, Astrid, Helmut Sigel, and Roland K. O. Sigel, eds. Metals in Biological Systems. CRC Press, 2000.

JOURNALS AND ARTICLES
Nanotechnology and Metal-Based Therapies:

- Jain, Prashant K., et al. "Gold Nanoparticles as Therapeutic Agents: Advances and Challenges." Chemical

Society Reviews, vol. 41, no. 7, 2012, pp. 2849-2864.

- Murphy, Catherine J., et al. "Gold Nanoparticles in Biology: Beyond Toxicity to Cellular Imaging." Accounts of Chemical Research, vol. 41, no. 12, 2008, pp. 1721-1730.

Antimicrobial Properties of Metals:

- Lemire, Joseph A., Joe J. Harrison, and Raymond J. Turner. "Antimicrobial Activity of Metals: Mechanisms, Molecular Targets, and Applications." Nature Reviews Microbiology, vol. 11, no. 6, 2013, pp. 371-384.
- Lansdown, A. B. G. "A Review of the Use of Silver in Wound Care: Facts and Fallacies." British Journal of Nursing, vol. 13, no. 6, 2004, pp. S6-S19.

Integrative Medicine:

- Maizes, Victoria, et al. "Integrative Medicine and Patient-Centered Care."

Explore: The Journal of Science and
Healing, vol. 5, no. 5, 2009, pp. 277-289.
- Rakel, David, and Nancy Faass.
  Integrative Medicine. Saunders, 2003.

ONLINE RESOURCES
World Health Organization (WHO):

> "Traditional, Complementary and Integrative Medicine." World Health Organization, 2021. https://www.who.int/health-topics/traditional-complementary-and-integrative-medicine

National Institutes of Health (NIH):

> "Nanotechnology and Human Health." National Institute of Environmental Health Sciences, 2021. https://www.niehs.nih.gov/research/supported/exposure/nano/index.cfm

PUBMED:
- "Gold Nanoparticles for Cancer Therapy." PubMed, 2021. https://pubmed.ncbi.nlm.nih.gov/

AMERICAN HOLISTIC HEALTH ASSOCIATION (AHHA):

- "Holistic Health and Wellness Resources." AHHA, 2021. https://ahha.org/

About
Dr. Constance
Santego

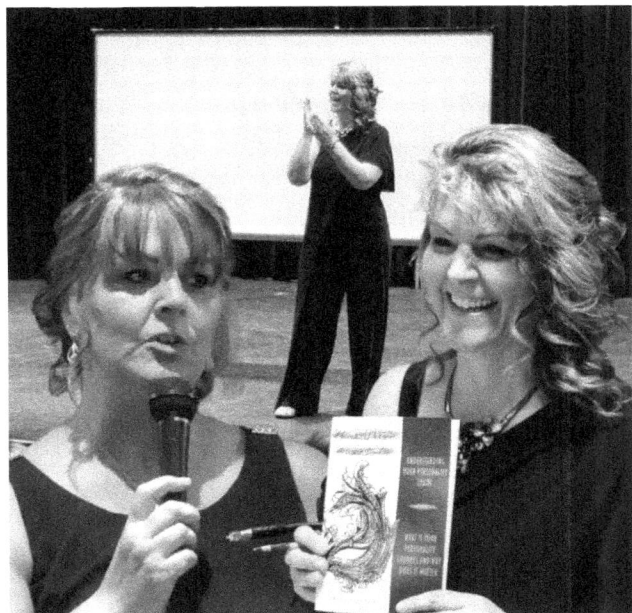

Dr. Constance Santego is a highly respected expert in the field of holistic health and spiritual healing, with over twenty-five years of experience teaching courses on these subjects. She has developed a deep understanding of the interconnectedness of the mind, body, and spirit in achieving overall well-being.

Dr. Santego holds a Ph.D. and Doctorate in Natural Medicine, which has provided her with a comprehensive understanding of alternative healing modalities and their application in promoting optimal health. Her educational background has equipped her with the knowledge to address health concerns from a holistic perspective, considering the physical, emotional, and spiritual aspects of an individual's well-being.

Throughout her career, Dr. Santego has been committed to sharing her knowledge and empowering others to take control of their health and healing. She has a unique ability to blend scientific research and traditional wisdom, creating a bridge between conventional and alternative medicine.

In addition to her expertise in various holistic practices, Dr. Santego is proficient in the field of Ring Therapy. This innovative approach combines the ancient wisdom of metals and their healing properties with modern muscle testing techniques to determine the optimal metal and finger placement for individual health concerns. Through her extensive research and practical application, Dr. Santego has developed a system that helps individuals achieve balance and well-being by wearing specific metal rings on designated fingers.

She also contributes her extensive knowledge in her "Secrets of a Healer" educational series, Dr. Santego draws upon her vast experience and expertise to captivate readers with her insights and teachings. She takes readers on a transformative journey, delving into the realms of holistic health, spirituality, and self-discovery. Through her writing, she aims to inspire individuals to tap into their own innate healing abilities and embrace a balanced and harmonious approach to well-being.

Dr. Santego's work has touched the lives of many, guiding them toward a more profound understanding of themselves and their connection to the world around them. Her series serves as a beacon of wisdom, offering practical tools and techniques for personal growth and transformation.

Overall, Dr. Constance Santego's blend of knowledge, experience, and passion makes her a captivating figure in the field of holistic health, spiritual healing, and ring therapy. Her contributions through teaching, writing, and her spellbinding series continue to inspire and empower individuals on their journeys toward well-being and self-discovery.

ALSO AVAILABLE

RING THERAPY PRACTITIONER CERTIFICATION PROGRAM

The ***Ring Therapy Practitioner Certification Program*** is a comprehensive course designed for individuals seeking to master the art of ring therapy for holistic healing. This program delves into the principles of Traditional Chinese Medicine (TCM), Ayurveda, and modern holistic practices, teaching you how to use metal rings to balance and enhance various body systems. You'll learn to apply these techniques effectively through detailed modules and hands-on practicum, providing personalized health solutions. Join us to gain valuable skills and become a certified practitioner, ready to help others achieve optimal health and well-being through ring therapy.

READ MORE:

https://constancesantego.ca/ring-therapy/

https://3jinn.com/courses/ring-therapy-practitioner-certification-program/

Email Notifications:

Go to our website to sign up and receive "Email Notifications" for upcoming Seminars, APPs, and other relevant information.

BOOKS
Ring Therapy: Guide to Healing and Balance

Trade Paperback ISBN: 978-1-990062-37-7
eBook ISBN 978-1-990062-38-4

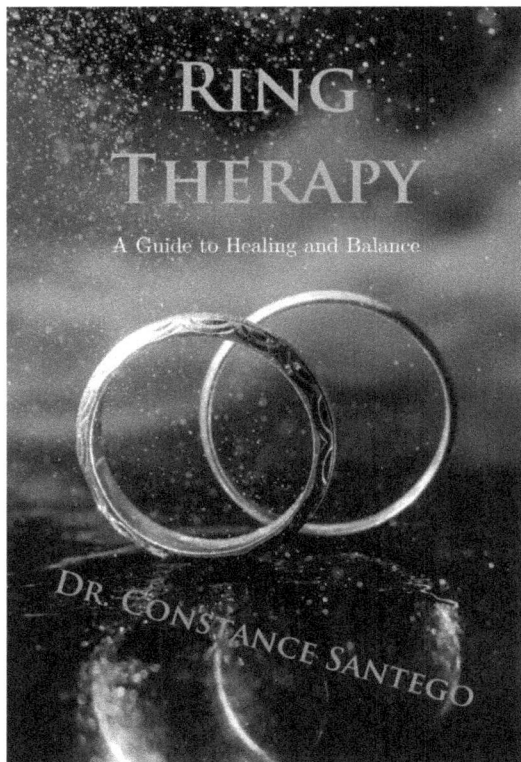

Secrets of a Healer...Magic of Muscle Testing

Trade Paperback ISBN: 978-0-9783005-3-1
eBook ISBN 978-0-9783005-5-5

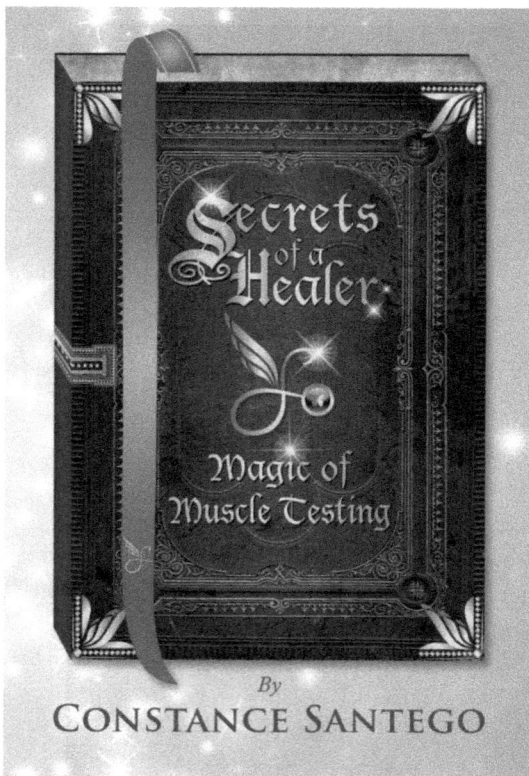

By
CONSTANCE SANTEGO

PLAY THE GAME *IKONA* – DISCOVER YOUR INNER GENIE

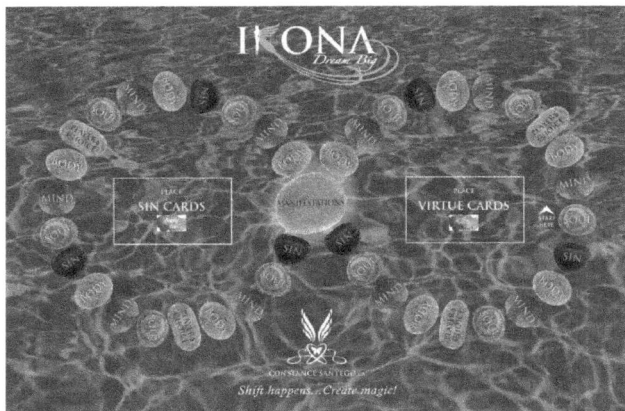

For additional information on

Constance Santego's wide range of Motivational Products, Coaching Sessions, Spiritual Retreats, Live Events and Educational Programs

Go to www.ConstanceSantego.ca

Follow on Instagram - Constance_Santego and Facebook - constancesantego

Subscribe and receive Free Information and Meditations on my YouTube Channel - Constance Santego

www.ingramcontent.com/pod-product-compliance
Lightning Source LLC
Chambersburg PA
CBHW060246030426
42335CB00014B/1609